Yoga for Beginners
The Ultimate Guide to Getting Started

By Nicole Townsend
Copyright © 2011

© 2011 by Nicole Townsend

ISBN-13: 978-1468190397

ISBN-10: 1468190393

All Rights Reserved. No part of this publication may be reproduced in any form or by any means, including scanning, photocopying, or otherwise without prior written permission of the copyright holder.

First Printing, 2011

Printed in the United States of America

Income Disclaimer

This book contains business strategies, marketing methods and other business advice that, regardless of my own results and experience, may not produce the same results (or any results) for you. I make absolutely no guarantee, expressed or implied, that by following the advice below you will make any money or improve current profits, as there are several factors and variables that come into play regarding any given business.

Primarily, results will depend on the nature of the product or business model, the conditions of the marketplace, the experience of the individual, and situations and elements that are beyond your control.

As with any business endeavor, you assume all risk related to investment and money based on your own discretion and at your own potential expense.

Liability Disclaimer

By reading this book, you assume all risks associated with using the advice given below, with a full understanding that you, solely, are responsible for anything that may occur as a result of putting this information into action in any way, and regardless of your interpretation of the advice.

You further agree that our company cannot be held responsible in any way for the success or failure of your business as a result of the information presented in this book. It is your responsibility to conduct your own due diligence regarding the safe and successful operation of your business if you intend to apply any of our information in any way to your business operations.

Terms of Use

You are given a non-transferable, "personal use" license to this book. You cannot distribute it or share it with other individuals.

Also, there are no resale rights or private label rights granted when purchasing this book. In other words, it's for your own personal use only.

Table of Contents

Yoga 101: Welcome to the World of Yoga............7
Myths and Truths of Basic Yoga..........................9
Pluses to Basic Yoga 13
Different Types of Yoga 17
Simple Warm-Up to Basic Yoga 21
Basic Yoga Exercise – Asana 25
Breathing for Yoga (Pranayama)......................35
Stop! Considerations before Beginning............37
Equipment for Beginners 41
Yoga in Losing Weight! 45
Expectations Beginner to Advanced Yoga.........49
FAQ's.. 51
Why Yoga?...53
Yoga and Stress 55
Yoga at Home and Away.....................................59
Yoga Class Expectations 65
How to Pose.. 71
Final Thoughts 83

Yoga 101: Welcome to the World of Yoga

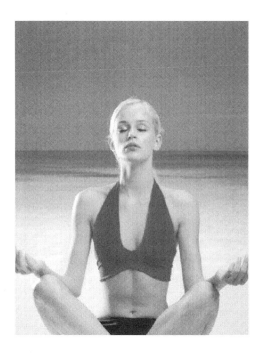

I'm sure you've got a vision in your head of what yoga is. And my guess is it involves a person the flexes like a pretzel, sitting on the floor with their legs crossed more than they should be, and likely in some sort of praying position with their hands. Of course they are chanting and in some sort of trance too. Am I right?
Well regardless, yoga is so much more and the great thing is that it's beneficial for people of all ages. And with yoga there is always progression, and the progression is at your pace!

Now let's have a gander at the beginnings of this powerful practice. Yoga comes from the language of Sanskrit, and literally refers to 'union'. The purpose of yoga is to balance your mind and body and search for pure and surreal self-enlightenment.

To implement this concept yoga marries moving, posing, breathing and relaxed meditative measures to achieve a healthy, balanced and full-filling life. Piece of cake right?

My Thoughts . . .
Actually Yoga makes me think of 'Yoda' from Star Wars, you know that cute little alien-type guy? But that has nothing to do with Yoga except maybe that he was wise and calm, so we'll leave it at that.
My attitude is you never know if you're going to like something unless you try! Time to step outside of your comfort zone and do something good for your mind and body!

No worries my friends because we are going to ease into this one pose at a time. And before you know it you'll have all the knowledge you need to confidently get yoga-ing!

Myths and Truths of Basic Yoga

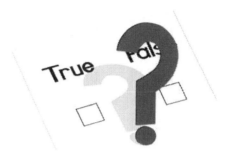

Myth: All Types Of Yoga Is Absolutely 100% Safe.
The problem here my friends, falls into the reason-ability factor. So if we are being completely truthful we can't say that all yoga is safe. This is where you need to use your noggin a little. If you haven't got up off the couch in a week and have just recovered from serious back surgery, and think you can go to your first 'expert' yoga class ever and successfully complete a 'downward dog' maneuver, you are going to bust yourself up.

The key is to ease into whatever sort of yoga class you are doing so that your body will get used to or warmed-up to the expectations these classes will have on it.
A little common sense and you'll do spectacularly!

Myth: Yoga Is A Fast Way To Drop Fat!
This is another tough one because with most yoga techniques you are looking to slow down your body, metabolism and all. Now this doesn't mean you won't

tone and strengthen your body and lose any weight. But losing it fast just isn't going to happen with yoga. Besides, losing weight effectively is a combination of eating well and exercising through building muscle and increasing your cardiovascular capacity. Need I say more?

Myth: All Yoga Instructors Are Top Of The Line!
I hate to burst your positive thinking bubble, but as with everything in life there are always those that seem to spoil the party! There's a bad bale in every wagon of hay if you will. It is important that you make certain your yoga instructor is qualified and the easiest way to do this is ask!

Find out how much experience they have and what sort of training courses they have taken to qualify them. If they tell you they just learned from other instructors and really don't have any credentials, no matter how 'hunky' they are, you should likely look for another class just to be safe!

'Hunky' isn't going to help you when you've put your back out because of using the wrong technique in your beginner yoga class! I feel the need for some positive right now, so here we go!

Truth: Yoga Will Make You Feel Spectacular!
I'm proud to report that yoga has been scientifically proven to de-stress you and boost your mood. In studies it has been successful in relieving depression and deterring it from starting in the first place. Regular yoga classes will also relax you and knock down your blood pressure numbers. It will get your endorphins running and this is going to naturally give you that 'feel good' feeling that is comparable to a runner's high.

A natural boost without being illegal and it last a whole lot longer without any crashing. What a great catch!

Truth: Yoga Will Better Your Sex Life! Bring It On!!!
Truth be told, yoga may be one of the best moves you can make to rev up the engines in your sex life. What happens is that yoga triggers your sex hormones to rise, particularly testosterone. Your brain waves are working overtime and they are engaged similarly to a newly 'in-love' couple.

Studies have proven the breathing techniques instigate sexual arousal. Some experiments were even done on married couples that were 'bored' in the bedroom. Concluding that after yoga sessions their bedrooms were just like Disneyland! With yoga you will have increased desire, confidence, arousal, orgasms and overall satisfaction of sex in general. And interestingly enough yoga helps men have better erections. All good when push comes to shove!

Truth: Yoga Is Spirituality
There has been debate that Yoga is a religion because it is closely related to Hinduism. Although this is true, yoga is not a religion in itself, but rather a sort of healing for the body and mind. This is definitely outside the controversial realm of religion.

My Thoughts . . .
Again you really need to be careful what you believe these days, except of course never question anything I say! (Just kidding!) We have so much information at our fingertips that it really can be overwhelming.

So what you need to do is make sure you use common sense when sifting through information on yoga truths and myths. If someone tells you that taking a yoga class where there is some chanting really equates to brainwashing you, then you need to question them. Simply because this only happens once in a while!

Follow your instincts and if you're not sure about something, just ask, then ask again. Make sure you get down to the root of any questions you might have so that you are venturing into the amazing world of yoga with truthful information!

Now it's time for us to have a look at a few of the positive benefits of getting your body moving to Yoga.

Pluses to Basic Yoga

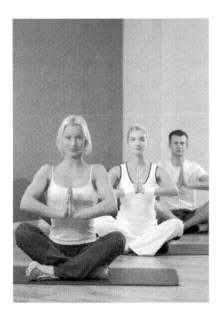

It's tough to know where to begin with the benefits you will get in practicing yoga. That said we're going to dive right in if you don't mind!

Yoga is going to:

-Massage The Organs Of Your Body – I think it's safe to say that yoga is just about the only 'exercise' out there that thoroughly massages and relaxes all of your internal organs, including the ones you don't even know exist! By internally relaxing your organs you are helping to improve function and deter negative energy from building up and translating into pain and disease.

-**Increase Your Flexibility** – Yoga will help your body to relax as a whole and this is going to encourage your muscles to engage and get active, when otherwise they would just sit still. Yoga isn't about seeing how far you can stretch but rather how well you can, if that makes sense to you. Slow and gentle wins the race with yoga.

-**Detoxify Your Body** – Your body is going to thank you for taking yoga sessions. Partly because yoga is going to help your muscles and organs relax and by massaging them yoga is naturally encouraging your body to flush out the harmful toxins or free radicals of the world that are accumulated in your system.

What this does is help to fill you full of energy, delay aging and bring back your desire to live life to the fullest, the spark if you will.

-**Naturally lubricate your ligaments, tendons and joints** – Rigorous research shows that various yoga positions strengthen and loosen specific ligaments and tendons of your body. Yoga instills calmness on you like no other and this seems to intensify the positive effects. So you really don't need to work as hard to stretch further, if that makes sense.

Yoga encourages harmony between your mind and body and in doing so it naturally helps you run better as a whole, joints and all!

-**Tone And Strengthen Your Muscles** – If you are just thinking about starting yoga, chances are you have some muscles you haven't used in a while. No worries my friend because yoga is going to gently stretch and strengthen your muscles, helping them to harden and take shape, giving you a shape you can't wait to show off!

-**Lowers Blood Pressure** – Yoga really does knock your blood pressure down a few notches. Through the gentle stretching motions of yoga you will improve your circulation and this is going to help more oxygenated blood flow through to your essential organs and supporting bodily systems. If you remove stress and relieve pressure, you are going to decrease your blood pressure!

-**Improves Your Respiratory Function** – As with your circulatory system, by attaining a lower respiratory ready you are showing that your lungs are working better. With the unique breathing techniques found in yoga you will learn to lower your respiratory rate, meaning your body is working less while being more productive.

-**Better Your Immunity** – Studies have indicated for years that regular yoga classes will help to strengthen your ability to resist the free radicals of the world. The free radicals are all the negatives in and around you that will cause harm to you mentally and physically. If your mind and body are stronger, you will be less likely to succumb to sickness. Yoga will help you build up your defenses and better you for it.

-**Improve Pain Tolerance** – Like it or not my friends; pain is a part of life. Whether you stub your toe on the door or have to deal with the chronic pain of migraines, improving your pain tolerance is a smart move. Yoga seems to tap into specific chemical that will actually help mask pain, leaving you less likely to notice it. This doesn't mean it isn't there but you have the ability to not focus on it, or work through it better.

Yoga allows you to tap into this and be better for it.
-**Fine Tunes Metabolism** – Now we aren't going to say that yoga lowers your metabolisms, but we will say that it helps to balance your metabolism and inhibit your hunger

cues from taking over. With routine yoga you will help your metabolism run more efficiently and when you are in control, you are less likely to add unwanted pounds.

My Thoughts . . .
Perhaps I'm a little one-sided, but for good reason. There are just so many positive benefits mentally and physically from taking yoga classes that it really tough to know where to begin!

Most of us, including me, don't really understand how powerful our mind is. It influences everything we do whether it's consciously or not. Sure yoga helps you relax, focus and think better, but it does so many other great things internally that we aren't even aware of. Just think of yoga as positive energy and you can't go wrong!

There are just so many benefits in getting your body moving with yoga. But it's time for us to move on to discuss, or rather my writing about, the different kinds of yoga out there.

Different Types of Yoga

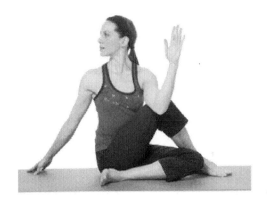

There are a variety of yoga disciplines out there and I don't want to get too confusing! So here is a list of 7 basic kinds of yoga with a brief explanation to get you started.

Bhakti Yoga
This translates in Hindu to realize God. It involves a spiritual journey that embraces love, and allows you to spiritually connect your mind and body.

Karma Yoga
This type of yoga translated means 'working with awareness'. It focuses on not viewing daily tasks as work, but rather as a means to increasing your awareness and tickling your senses. It consciously helps you connect with your life situations, whether you are wrestling, cleaning toilets or tending to your garden.

Jnana Yoga
This is recognized as the yoga of true knowledge. It's based on the unique thinking of non-dualism, a Hindu philosophy. Basically looking into the truth of what we are experiencing and of who we really are.

Raja Yoga
This kind of yoga is also known as 'Royal Yoga'. It's a part of all yogis, the thinking behind it more complex than any of the other yoga disciplines of today. It focuses on the advantages of meditating for self-realization through spirit and expansion of your thinking.

Mantra Yoga
This yoga discipline uses the science of sound. It's a metaphysical philosophy that traces out the path of evolution and the journey itself. Think of Mantra yoga as the vessel that carries you across the lake of thoughts.

Tantra Yoga
Tantra yoga will help you dissolve limitations and transform this new found energy into internal strength, power and energy for internal transformation and healing. It recognizes wealth and enjoyment and looks to help you balance your inner and outer self.

Hatha Yoga
This describes the physical practice of yoga. Hatha is used to describe the basic and gentle sessions with no

flow between various poses. This offers often slow and controlled stretching and breathing sessions.

Wow! That's a whole lot of different types of yoga, and that's just brushing the surface!

My Thoughts . . .
Now if you feel like a boat out of water right now, don't sweat it, because you won't feel that way for long! The idea is to do as I did and get uncomfortable to get comfortable. Don't push yourself and concentrate on these different kinds of yoga one kind at a time. Before you know it you will be the one instructing the classes!

Now let's have a look at getting started.

Simple Warm-Up to Basic Yoga

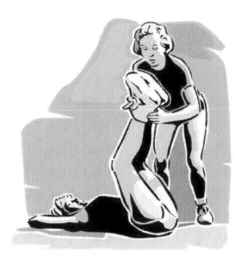

For any type of exercise it is incredibly important for you to warm up. This is especially true if you are just testing out the waters in a beginner's yoga class. Yeah you!

Chances are pretty good that if you happen to arrive early to your session, you are going to see your classmates engaging in a variety of warm-up exercises. You may feel like a knob because you really don't know what to do and this is where I can help you. Read on my friend!

Take note that most beginner yoga classes are going to warm you up in the actual class, but it can't hurt to get your juices flowing even before this happens.

Pelvic Tilts

This one is a pretty simple exercise to get your core loose. Just lie down on your back with your knees bent and hands at your sides. All you do is gently press your back against the floor and release. This is going to help get your blood circulating and kick in some of those 'feel good' drugs you have stored in your system!

Eagle Arms
Sit down comfortably with your arms in front of you at a 90 degree angle. Cross your elbows over one another while crossing your hands as well and clasping your hands together. This will stretch you nicely across the shoulder blades. Repeat this by crossing your elbows and hands the other way.

Cat Stretch
These are great for loosening your spine. Get on your hands and knees comfortable. Now push your head down towards the floor while arching your back up high towards the sky. Hold this for a ten count and then release back down while pulling your head up and pushing your navel toward the ground. Repeat.

Child's Pose
This is a great stretch for your hips and thighs. Just kneel down on the mat with your chin touching the mat and arms outstretched in front of you. Make sure your movements are gentle because you don't want to pull anything

These are just a few basic stretches you can perfect just in case you've got a few minutes before your yoga session begins.

My Thoughts . . .
Honestly all the different types of yoga stretches really confused me at first, and it still does sometimes. So

don't worry if you aren't quite familiar with them yet. The best method of learning about them is to experience them, not all at once though!

Start with one and as you get comfortable add to your arsenal. Before you know it you'll know them all!

Moving on . . .it's time for Asana!

Basic Yoga Exercise – Asana

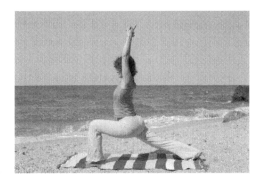

Asana refers to body positions in yoga lingo. It also indicates the place and form your body is in. Don't worry because I'm not going to get too technical on you here or I'm just going to end up confusing myself too! Now pay attention because we are going to get started now.

The thinking behind yoga exercise in general is that you have various joints in your body that need regular movement and lubrication, agreed? Well the food you fill your tummy with provides the lubrication and various other activities give your body the movement.

What happens is that life takes a toll on you and most of your joints end up being used too much and this often creates issues later in life. A point in which we discover our body isn't really invincible!

Chin up my friend because Yoga will help you restore and strengthen your joints and it's the yoga movements

that are going to help you get healthier mentally and physically. Make sense?
Now onto a few of the yoga positions for asana with a little insight tossed in! Aren't you excited?
And please note that yoga exercises are all about focus. You need to be aware of body position, breathing, rhythm and mind control to start (not the hypnotizing kind!).

Cobra Pose

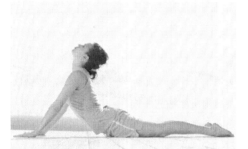

I'm sure you've heard of this one before. It helps to strengthen your lower back, spine, chest area, lungs and middle.

Fish Pose

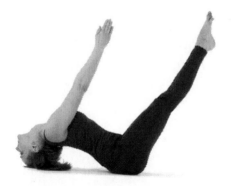

This one is also called Matsyasana and no, it's not smelly! It looks to benefit your chest muscles, upper back and neck area.

Cat Pose

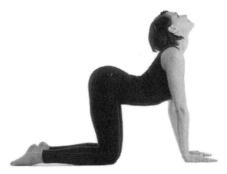

This one we mentioned previously if you were paying attention, which I'm sure you were. It helps tremendously in getting rid of any tightness in your spine and back.

Bridge Pose

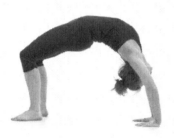

A Bridge Pose is also referred to as Setu Bandhasana. This maneuver will warm your chest, shoulders, spine, neck and breathing.

Child Pose

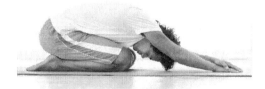

Balasana will help to elongate or stretch out your back area, hips and thighs. This is a really relaxing move that reminds you of parts you don't usually use!

Hero Pose

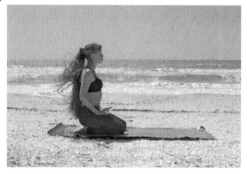

This one has a second name called Virasana. It will relieve pressure in your knees, legs and thighs and will also help to smooth out digestion. Bet you didn't see that one coming!

Boat Pose

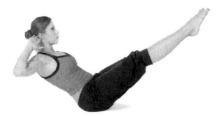

This yoga move will help in your quest to build strength in your hips, abs and spine area. This is very important in maintaining a strong core.

Eagle Pose

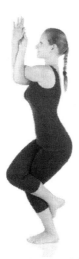

This one sounds really cool. And it looks to help improve your balance and coordination, while stretching out your back area, hips and thighs specifically.

Lotus Pose

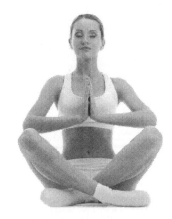

This neat move will stimulate energy in your pelvic area and spine. It will also stretch your knees and ankles.

Plow Pose

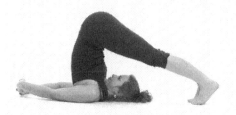

This pose makes me think of farming! It looks to build strength and versatility in your spine, abs area, and neck.

Chair Pose

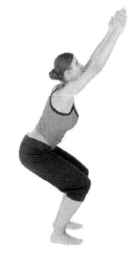

Have a seat without the chair my friend. This move will work to build strength and stability in your legs, arms, spine and it will help wake up your diaphragm.

Downward-Facing Dog Pose

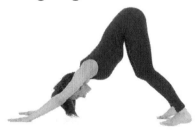

Now this particular pose is a popular one you may have heard of before. This asana will stretch out your legs and shoulders and will help to settle your brain.

Half Lord of the Fish Pose

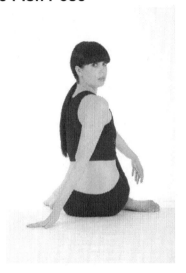

Now that's a mouthful! This maneuver will work to strengthen your spine, while stretching out your hips, thighs, shoulders and neck area.

Now get out there and do them! It really is important to ensure you have proper technique and are comfortable to concentrate while performing your yoga asana. As a beginner make sure you get a qualified instructor to show you the ropes. It won't be long before you will extend your knowledge even further and shortly after will be practicing your asana in the line waiting for the movies!

My Thoughts . . .
Now these poses may be intimidating at first. At least the names are! But you will soon warm up to them. Take your time and concentrate on them one at a time when

you are testing the waters. And don't be afraid to try practicing them at home to get familiar.
You know what they say, practice makes perfect! Or in my case it just makes me a little bit better!

Don't hold your breath because we're on to the next issue at hand.

Breathing for Yoga (Pranayama)

Without breathing you would be in big trouble. But did you know that 'how' you breathe helps dictate how well your body will run, what sort of health challenges you will face and how long you will live?

Yoga believes strongly that the more 'aware' you are of your breathing and the better that you 'control' it; the better off you'll be mentally, physically and emotionally. Guess what? They are right.

Now we aren't going to go too deep here but we will get to the bottom of why breathing 'better' is so important. Pranayama means 'life force' and 'control'.

Yoga breathing is practiced when you are performing asana and it helps you understand the importance of diaphragmatic and thoracic breathing. Of course there are basic and advanced breathing techniques but understanding this basic concept will help you to grasp the concept quickly and maybe even tune in better on the big picture.

With basic Prayanama puraka or breathing; it encourages your body to load your lungs with fresh air. Holding your breath will help increase your internal temperature and helps your body to increase the ability to absorb oxygen. Rechalk or exhalation will force your diaphragm to head back to its regular position and all of the impure air is sent out of your body through the contraction of your intercostal muscles. Are you following?

These are the basic concepts of Prayanama. And Prayanama massages your abdominal area helps tone the organ in your body. And by paying special attention to your bodily organs you are going to open your energy channels and help your body run more efficiently as a whole.

What's important to note is that Pranayama is dependent on the exact ratio of retention, exhalation and breathing in. This is something you can always work on and improve. Quite inspiring don't you think?

My Thoughts . . .
It's funny how very little we think about something so important as breathing! You don't breathe and you die! Luckily we have a backup system that makes breathing automated or we would be in big trouble!
And it's interesting to note that practicing your breathing really does make a difference in your energy levels and mindset. But the only way you are likely going to believe this is to try it. So get to it!

Stop! Considerations before Beginning

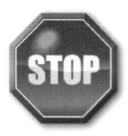

Now you may have in your head that yoga is all gentle and relaxing, and it is. But whenever you are venturing into any sort of new exercise regimen you need to make sure you are aware of a few things.

Consideration One
It is really important to ensure you are learning yoga from a qualified instructor. If you don't you could end up learning asana incorrectly and this could lead to serious injury; not to mention the fact that you wouldn't be developing a solid base from which to build your yoga from.

All you have to do is ask my friend. Make sure you see where they've been qualified to teach beginner yoga, their experience and any schooling and credentials they possess. Ask around too because that definitely can't hurt. Just because they aren't hard on the eyes doesn't mean they are good even a qualified yoga instructor!

Consideration Two
Make certain you are signing up for a beginner class and not an elite one. Ensure that you are clear to whomever you're talking to that you have no prior yoga experience and are looking to get involved in learning yoga in a beginner class.

Unfortunately there are some people that will try and convince you that they have a 'specialty' class that you will do just fine in, but it's not really for beginners. Don't fall for it. You are a beginner and you need a beginner class.

Consideration Three
Check out the numbers of the class you are thinking of attending. If possible you really don't want to start in a class that if too full, or one that only has one or two people for that matter. A moderate size will work best because there are a few others to learn from and this won't make you feel too awkward to start.

Consideration Four
You need to know your schedule and our natural energy pattern. By this I mean that if you are completely exhausted after dinner and know that you are just going to want to hit the hay, don't sign up for your yoga session then!

If you have most of your energy in the morning and know that your appointments for work don't start until about 11 each day, then a 9 am yoga class will work perfect for you.

The idea is that you need to make sure you sign up for a class that you are going to have energy for and that you are going to be able to commit to on a routine basis.

Consideration Five
Make sure you talk with your potential instructor and trust your gut. You need to feel comfortable with your instructor and it's important that you feel positive energy from them, like they are excited about teaching yoga.

These are key factors in determining how much you are going to enjoy your yoga classes and how much you will learn. Monkey see, monkey do. If you 'feel' and 'see' that your instructor loves what they do and are excited to help you learn, it will be smooth sailing into port.

Consideration Six
Now you may be all excited about the idea of learning yoga but don't forget about your budget. Make sure you inquire as to the cost of the classes before you sign on the dotted line. Ask about discounts or any specials that may be offered to save you a few dollars.

The fact is; that it will be pretty tough to enjoy and be relaxed in your beginner yoga class if you are stressed about your money situation.

It really is a key point that you take a little bit of extra time to make sure you find the right yoga class for you. Trust me; it pays to find a great class sand great instructor from which to build!

My Thoughts . . .
It's also important to note that you check with your doctor before starting any yoga sessions. This is just a precaution so that I don't get into any hot water! But really folks;

life is full of surprises and it's important to make sure that you don't experience any nasty ones if you can help it. Be safe not sorry and scoot in to have a doctor give you a once over so that you can get started with your yoga with a clean bill of health!

Now let's have a look at what you need to start!

Equipment for Beginners

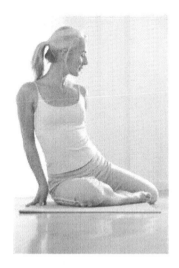

Of course with the concept of yoga you are supposed to be relaxed and calm and to help with this you really need the right equipment. Now don't fret because you really don't need a whole lot of equipment to start. In fact make sure you inquire but many facilities will provide you with what you need for a beginner class.

You may find it nice to be using your own stuff. It really isn't pleasant to think about using mats that other people have sweat all over!

Here are a few things you might like to purchase:
Yoga Mat
It's not hard to guess that this is usually the first item that new yoga enthusiasts purchase. Makes sense because it is the main piece of equipment used.

Now you will want to buy a high quality yoga mat that doesn't shift around while you are moving. This means you shouldn't opt for the cheapies at the Dollar Store my friend! It needs to be fairly thick and comfy to sit on.

You'll also need to consider the length and make sure that you aren't selling yourself short. If you are really tall it's especially important that you pay attention to this factor. You'd be surprised how many people make it to their first yoga class and find out they have a really nice mat that's just too small!

You should be able to lay outstretched on your mat without your head, hands or feet hanging off. Unroll it and do a lay-down test if need be before you buy it.

Yoga Blocks
Yoga blocks most often are composed of foam-like material. But they can also be made from wood. They are recommended for helping to provide relief from some of the pressures that result from various stand up poses. As well, they are great for any positions you are implementing where your head or hands are on the floor. This may not make sense to you right now but it will after your first class!

Yoga Blankets
Yoga blankets have numerous different versatile uses. When you are calming yourself with meditation, they are great for helping to make the situation more real by pulling it over your head. This really is just better for your concentration as a whole.

Blankets are also used to help with your stability when you are holding specific poses. This is especially beneficial when you are just starting out, that's you! And when you are choosing a blanket make sure it makes you smile and brighten your mood. A bright color often helps with this or one with a really neat design. It also needs to be soft to the touch and comfortable and not itchy to lie on. Don't try to get by with an itchy old bath towel because that just won't cut it!

Mediation Cushions
Meditation cushions are excellent for keeping your bottom comfortable when you are in a sitting position. Of course there are a diverse range from which you can choose. You just need to ensure you buy one that works with your body type, not too big or too small, and that it is durable. Buying a cheap cushion means you are going to have to buy it again, your choice!

I think that's just about it. Equipment really is an integral part of getting yourself set properly for your first yoga experience. You need to gather your equipment prior to starting class so that you really do benefit fully from the yoga classes. A little bit of investment also doesn't hurt to help sway you into getting to class, because you do have a little bit invested in it!

My Thoughts . . .
With most things in life you can get by with just about any kind of equipment. We used to skate on the pond with sticks tied to the bottom of our boots! But if you have half decent equipment you are more likely to enjoy your new activity
.
There isn't a whole lot of cost to get started with yoga, so do what you have to so that you have at least a good mat and towel to start. Just because you are worth it!

Now there aren't too many people out there that are 100% satisfied with their body. Most of these particular people want to lose weight. Yoga can help you with this . . . read on!

Yoga in Losing Weight!

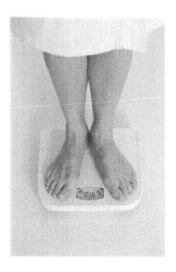

Most of us have tried this, that and everything to try and lose weight. We waste time yo-yoing back and forth depending on the season at hand. Sound familiar? What if I were to tell you that yoga can help you drop that fat for good? Would you be excited and want to know more?

Part of the problem with losing weight is that we often set ourselves up to fail, but making 'temporary' changes that we know aren't going to stick, and by calling it a 'diet!' In order to lose weight and keep it off you need to make healthy changes in your lifestyle and stick with it and yoga can help you do just that.

If you want to look sexy in your new string biking, yoga is the answer. Research suggests that individuals that have maintained regular yoga classes for more than 4 years actually gained less weight as they got older. And to top that stat, people that did yoga sessions for more than 4 years ended up losing weight over a 10 year span. Pretty great news don't you think?

And it's not just the physical exercise in yoga classes that help burn off fat. Experts agree that your mind needs to be on board with all of this if you are going to lose weight and keep it off for good.

To back this theory there is a whole bunch of different programs out there that combine various physical activities with mindful thinking in order to lose weight. All of these programs dictate that people need to weight their thoughts of food against their emotional feeling. Things like anxieties, fear, anger or boredom, to ensure they are chomping down for the right reasons.

Instead of using high fat foods to satisfy your emotions, you can opt to provide relief by learning to settle your head with relaxation techniques like deep breathing and meditation. By being attune to your mind a little more, you are less likely to make poor health choices.

The techniques you learn in yoga in various poses, to stay focused on your breathing and sense of calm, you can transfer over to use when you are dealing with food issues. You will become more aware of your senses and your body as a whole. What you need and don't need and this thought alone is going to help you lose weight in the big picture.

It is fair to say that there are many out there that don't believe yoga can help with weight loss. If you are eating right, focus on the things you should and stick with your yoga sessions, expanding your knowledge and ability, you can shed pounds and more importantly keep them off!

The fact is that done correctly, yoga can help you build muscle and doing this is going to help your body run more efficiently as a whole. Increasing your natural metabolism and this means that even when you are taking a snooze you are going to be burning more calories than if you just spent your life lounging on the couch!

The continuous posing in yoga will also get your heart rate up will help to build your endurance levels, the key in helping to get rid of fat. Combining this with a healthy lifestyle in general and you will lose weight and that part is a good inevitable!

My Thoughts . . .
Yoga can help you lose weight with the right combination of eating well and maintaining a positive and healthy lifestyle. But if you are heading into yoga as a means to drop a whole bunch of fat quickly, that's just not going to happen. Why? Well because there isn't enough intense muscle building and cardiovascular activity.
You are best to use yoga in combination with other more strenuous exercise sessions to drop fat quickly.

Expectations Beginner to Advanced Yoga

Beginner yoga is all about understanding the benefits of yoga and the various styles practiced. Learning the basics of controlling your mind and how to focus is the key in understanding how to become better attuned with your body.

Of course here is also where you will learn how to breathe and perfect the basic yoga poses. Each session gets more comfortable in your skin and thereby improving your emotional and physical well-being with each asana.

With time and experience you will gain confidence and graduate in practicing humility in advanced yoga. You can expect to strive towards creating harmony within your body, mind and soul. It's for people familiar with yoga concepts and techniques, and gradual process of expanding upon your ethics, morals and concentration knowledge.

You can expect to strengthen your mind, enabling you to do surreal things like walking through fire. Not that you will do this, but the idea in advanced yoga is that you will gain incredible mental power that will enable you to do what you once thought to be impossible.
As your mind powers strengthen you will unite further with the universe around you.

My Thoughts . . .
You will know when it's time to move past beginning yoga classes. It's not systematic where after 10 classes you move onto the next level. Yoga takes into consideration your dedication, ability, desire and understanding of beginner yoga concepts, strategies, breathing and asana before looking to advance. It's not a race, and isn't measured by time, as much as the mindset and comprehension.

FAQ's

Can I do yoga during menstruation?
This question has mixed reviews because some experts feel you should relax during your menstruation days, but others think you should practice with limitation. The best answer is to do what you feel is best for you and your body!

How many days a week should I practice yoga?
Well, real yogis practice every day, but that's not usually practical for most people. It is something that you need to find time to do fairly routinely though, so the minimum is really three days per week.

If I have health issues can I still take yoga?
Absolutely! Of course check with your doctor and make sure your instructor is aware of any limitations you might have. Yoga will actually help release some of your negative energy and help you feel better about yourself as a whole regardless of your health issues!

Do guys take yoga?
Of course! Now they may not be the majority, but this doesn't mean they don't take it and aren't enjoying it. If you'd feel better why not bring a male friend along with you? The key is to not let your sexual orientation limit you!

Can you be too old to take yoga?
No, you can't! Experts agree that any sort of exercise is better than no exercise regardless of your age. In fact the older you get the more important it is for you to keep

your body moving. If you don't you will start to cease up and may end up in a position where you are limited in your movements. Yoga will help you to avoid this!

When is the best time to practice?
The best time really is in the morning. But I understand this doesn't work for everyone. So anytime is better than nothing my friend!

My Thoughts . . .
There are just so many different questions people have about starting yoga. Just never be afraid to ask! I'm sure you've heard before that the only stupid question is the question not asked. Well it's absolutely true!

Why Yoga?

Well there really is no quick answer to this question because none of us think the same. This happens to be a good thing if you think about it! How about saying the main reason you should take yoga is because it leaves you feeling spectacular? Does that work?

Your mind, body and spirit get healthier through yoga by learning new postures, breathing techniques and meditation exercises. With yoga you can relax and tune out all the stresses life serves up daily simultaneously.

Now if you have any chronic health conditions or regular aches and pains, yoga will help you. It can help control arthritic, anxieties, and back pain. Yoga will also lower blood pressures, decrease depression, reduce headaches and decrease the risks of heart disease. Add to this the fact that yoga can:

- Build strength and stamina
- Tone muscles and improve cardiovascular capacity
- Get rid of annoying stresses and tension
- Improve your self-esteem
- Get rid of fat for good
- Help better your concentration and ability to create
- Better circulation
- Improve your immune system
- Calm and relax you

Sounds pretty good to start! Although these are all just topical benefits of taking regular yoga classes. Yoga really is a spiritual practice that was founded in India thousands of years ago. Yoga actually means 'union' in Sanskrit. This is a union of your body and mind. That is what yoga is trying to accomplish, even in the non-believers!

Ancient beliefs say you will achieve true happiness with the union of divine consciousness. Each practice of yoga is a branch trying to reach this ultimate goal of true happiness, inside and out. A smile is not only from your lips. For example, with Hatha yoga, breathing and various postures will help relax you, cleanse your mind, spirit and physical body so that this yogi can find union.

Pranayama breathing will help clear the energy channels within the universe, allowing blockages to dissipate and for this energy to gain power, effectiveness and momentum.

Yoga is not an act of enlightenment but rather a process in which you strive to gain pure energy and find balance. By peeling away the layers of emotions, conditions and sensations and you will find out who you really are. By striving for greater awareness you will become more sensitive and be able to unblock anything that is keeping you from finding your place.

Basically yoga will help you to gain control of yourself. It will help clear your mind and strengthen your body and allow you to discover and be happy with whom you really are.

Yoga and Stress

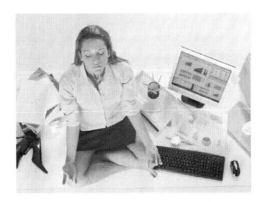

Life as we know it is often swallowed whole by stress whether we choose to admit it or not. Your life is loaded with deadlines, hassles, frustrations and complications.

Unfortunately what happens is over time we accept these harmful stresses as normal and adapt. This can manifest into serious issue over time.

Not to say that some stress isn't a good thing, because it is. Let's just say it keeps you on your toes and reminds us we are alive and kicking. But the majority of the time the stresses you and I are dealing with are slowing breaking us down, consciously or not.

If you are constantly trying to function under stress, this will affect your body and mind negatively. Sort of like swimming with a ten pound weight around your middle.

Sure you are ok to start and have no issues swimming. But over time this will literally weigh you down so that you just can't swim that last ten meters of the race.

Recognizing stress is the key in releasing it.

Stress is just a natural physical response to events that upset you or cause alarm. It is that good old 'fight or flight' response. Stress is the method in which your body tries to protect you. To help you stay focused and aware, ready to deal with whatever is in front of you.
How you respond to stress is important. Calm and controlled works best, but isn't always possible.

So what's important is that you do whatever you can to find a method that works for you to release stress in general. Get rid of the drama and worry and replace it with relaxed happiness.

And this is where yoga fits in because it is spectacular for your mind, body and soul.

Here are a few of the benefits of yoga with regards to managing your stress.

Did you that Yoga dates back over 5000 years ago and was effectively practiced for self-development? Classical yoga was inclusive of ethical disciplines, breathing, control and specific positions.

People are seeing that yoga is helping people be more productive, creative, happier and healthier. And yoga helps you to tune into your body and get things under control for lack of a better term. This is what reduces and releases your stress, whether it's circumstantial or in general.

The following are positive advantages of practicing yoga

on a regular basis and these are going to contribute directly towards stress reduction:

* sleeping better
* lower cortisol levels
* bettering medical conditions
* improved sense of self-worth
* looking and feeling better
* stronger body physically
* stronger and more intuitive mind
* lower heart rate - means heart works less
* lower anxiety levels
* less depression

All of these factors will help you become one with your body, sending stress packing and enabling yourself to start clearing the clutter and focus on the positive. How does that sound?

With yoga you are going to satiate your needs psycho-somatically (love that word!) and physically. And finding this strong balance is only going to make you a better you.

It's pretty hard to argue the fact that yoga is going to benefit you PERIOD. And when it comes to relieving and helping teach you how to avoid stress in the future, it's limitless.

I think it's time for you to get working on your downward dog!

My Thoughts . . .

Anything you can do to help get stress out of your system is a great thing. Stress will eat you up and spit you out if you let it. The problem is by the time we stop ignoring this fact, it's often too late.

The best time to act is now and what better way than through experimenting and learning the limitless world of relaxing and invigorating yoga.

You can get your mind and body into fabulous shape while you're having fun. Focusing on bettering yourself on all levels and kicking stress in the gut while you're doing this.

Sounds like a pretty sound option to me!

Now we are going to skip over to looking at the versatility of yoga!

Yoga at Home and Away

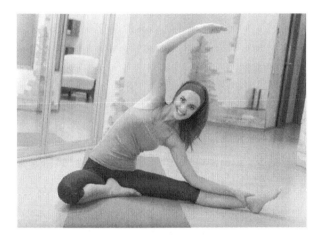

Yoga is something that you can take with you anywhere you go. If you're too busy to find a class you can easily do it in the comfort of your own home at any level. If you happen to be traveling, with a little preparation you can take it on the road with you no problem.

And it's not like you've got to throw a bike or treadmill into your backpack my friend! The reason is because very little, if any equipment is required.

I must caution you though especially if you are a beginner, that you do this safely. Don't just 'think' you can jump right into it without warming your body up and understand what your limitations are. If you try this you may put yourself out literally for a few months!

Start off slow and steady and you will win the race with yoga.

Here are a few thoughts that will help you to do yoga at home or abroad.

MAKE SPACE

This is important because you will need an uncluttered area with just enough space for you to do different yoga poses. This space will need to be calm and quiet and safe. Meaning no wet floors you could slip on or other objects lying around randomly.

And you don't need a whole lot of space. There's even plenty if you are staying in a hotel room.

EQUIPMENT BASICS

Now you don't have to have a heart attack here because your equipment can literally fit in your backpack. A simple yoga mat is something you should probably invest in.

They aren't very much money and you can get a thin one that rolls up tight and light, especially if you are taking it traveling. At home you may want to buy a couple blocks and a strap for modifications, but you really don't need that off the top.

Keep in mind this is the very basics, just a start. You can even get by if worse comes to worse without a yoga mat, although having one is really a good thing!

SAFETY FIRST

As mentioned previously it is incredibly important that you

have the area clear of clutter than you are going to be posing in. The last thing you need is to lose your footing because of a loose piece of paper or toy on the floor and injure yourself indefinitely.

Look around you before starting and do a double take, just in case. It could save who a whole bucket or aggravation!

PICK A STYLE OF YOGA

Are there lots of different yoga styles to choose from? Absolutely! Be happy about that because now you know you're going to find one that suits you perfectly!

The most common of course is Hatha. And your best bet is to choose one, experiment with it, and try one or two more just to figure out what style fits you like a glove.

INSTRUCTION

Of course having a few yoga sessions under your belt with a qualified instructor is invaluable in the big picture. They will answer any questions you might have, inspire you, ensure your technique is correct and give you pointers to make your yoga sessions more productive and enjoyable.

Even if you are doing yoga at home, taking one or two sessions prior certainly doesn't hurt. It's not a must though because if you inform yourself, you can do fabulously on your own to start.

The choice is yours and you need to do what's best for you.

TAKE THE INITIATIVE

Even if you are a busy body it's important to take the bull by the horns and do a little research. Information is knowledge and the more you know the better decisions you can make for you in anything you do, not just your yoga adventures.

You can read books, surf the net, buy a few magazines and just talk with friends that yoga. Doors of opportunity will open up for you and the confidence you gain with the information you are gathering will do wonders for you.

DON'T MAKE EXCUSES

We are creatures of habit and when trying something new it's just too easy to quit and jump back into our comfort zone of stoic pattern. Don't let this happen. Give yourself time to get used to your new yoga routine. And instead of finding a reason not to get your session in, look for ways to make it happen.

Just because you're planning to head to the beach early tomorrow doesn't mean you can't get a quick 20 minute yoga session in. Plan to either do it before you leave or maybe even at the beach!

There are endless options and changing things up keeps it interesting and better yet keeps your mind and body guessing!

EASY ON YOURSELF

Slow and steady really does win the race. DO NOT jump into yoga, particularly if you've never done it before.

Be smart and start slow. Make sure you ease yourself into it, one step at a time. Rushing will accomplish nothing and yoga is not about what you know, but rather what you are learning. It's a constant learning process and you are attempting to open your body and mind up, and this will happen when it should!

Most importantly you need to respect your body and listen to what it is telling you. Yoga is a learning process and you are going to be delighted with each class!

MOOD IS IMPORTANT

It is really important that you are able to focus when practicing yoga. And setting the ambiance is a very key point here. Many will play soft and gentle music in the background in order to get into the right mood.

You need to do whatever is necessary to bring your mind to a neutral state and set your worries aside. Set yourself up for success my friend and you will reap the rewards ten times!

MEDITATION

Regardless of where you are actually practicing yoga, meditation is a key component. Yoga is purposefully supporting meditation. Meditation will help you to relax your mind and get the most out of your yoga session.

Sure you can do yoga without meditation but that's like ordering a sundae without the cherry. It's just not the same.

Do yourself a favor. Find a comfortable position and take

a few minutes to meditate before you get into your yoga movements. You will benefit mentally and physically from it tremendously.

Trust me on this one!

My Thoughts . . .

There really is no reason to not find a few minutes to get your yoga in, no matter where you are. Yoga is incredibly versatile, with little equipment, and you can do it easily at home or when traveling.

All you've got to do is to commit to making it happen and it will. And it's just so tremendously beneficial for you, even if you are only able to squeeze 20 minutes in. That's 20 minutes more than you had.

You are important and you need your mind and body in tip-top condition to serve you well. Yoga will help you with this. Time for you to make sure it happens don't you think?

How about looking into to what to expect in a yoga session?

Yoga Class Expectations

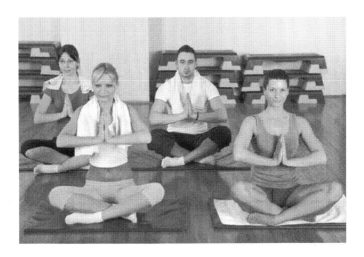

Clear your head of what you may be thinking about your first yoga class. You aren't going to walk in and the instructor is going to expect you to twist just like a pretzel. That won't happen until the second class . . .just kidding!

Relax.

A good instructor is going to work your body through a series of sequences that are going to get you ready for the posing, while making sure you aren't going to overdo it and injure yourself.

Here are a few things to expect.

LEARNING TO GET CENTERED

One of the first things you will do in your class is to learn to get centered. You can do this through breathing exercising, just sitting down or meditating.

This is where you will learn to focus on you and set your own personal goals for each session. Look at it as you would a five minute time out to get ready to start another task or head in another direction.

LOOSEN THOSE LIMBS
Of course warming your body up is incredibly important when partaking in any sort of physical activity. That's right! I said any activity requiring physical exertion.

Specific poses like the Cat Cow will help to loosen your shoulder and neck area, stimulate your circulation and get your body ready for a few more physical challenges.

And it doesn't hurt to do a little bit of light stretching, jumping jacks, or running on the spot before you even get to class. This will give you a head start on the warming up process and a jump on getting yourself into that yoga mode.

SALUTE THE SUN

Sun Salutations are a series of twelve movements that happen quickly. They will help to get your body warmed up and maybe even breaking a bit of a sweat. Indication your body is ready for more.

POSES ON YOUR FEET

Next up you can expect poses on your feet. The Warrior and Triangle poses help to strengthen and align your muscles, while using focus, endurance and balance. All of which will keep you moving forward.

GET BALANCED

Now you may well move into some balancing poses where the goal is to try not to let your feet hit the floor. Be graceful and powerful. The Eagle and Tree will help you gain control of your balance and focus, while you relax.

Have patience because this takes time to master but each time you will get closer to reaching your goals.

RIGHT-SIDE-UP

Here you will work on lifting your legs while you are literally upside down. This helps to improve your balance, while not putting the entire work load onto your arms.

Challenging yet rewarding!

BACKBENDS

Next you may expect some backbends. These will help to energize you by opening your chest and stimulating your adrenal glands.

SIMPLE TWISTS

These can really fall anywhere in the class as they will help to loosen you up and release pressure from your spine area.

Think of this as a cleansing moment, toxins beware!

SIT ON IT

Poses while you are seated are going to help relax your nervous system and set you up for relaxation. Examples are the Cobbler pose or the Pigeon pose.

SHOULDER STAND

The shoulder stand helps to renew your whole body. You'll have your shoulders, elbow and head on the floor, simultaneously while your butt and legs stretch gently towards the ceiling.

This rests your heart while getting your blood flowing nicely.

Often you can expect to do this with the Plow. This is where you'll slowly lower your legs to the ground behind your head.

LIE STILL

Next, the Corpse pose works perfectly. Here you will let your body completely relax into the floor, while calming your head. You are in total relaxation.

Finally you may expect to bow or chant 'namaste' or 'om'. This tells your teacher and fellow classmates that you've had an excellent class.

My Thoughts . . .

Trying anything new can do a number on your nerves; which is exactly the opposite of what you want to accomplish with yoga.

Knowing what sort of things to expect with your first session will definitely help to take the edge off and give you and edge on the other beginners joining you.

Time to get uncomfortable to get comfortable and enjoy your first yoga class!

Now we'll look into a few detailed poses:

How to Pose

Here we are going to look at different yoga asanas or poses and how to do them correctly.

THE CORPSE

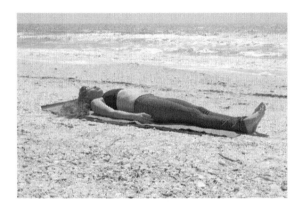

This is a relaxation pose and it may look easier than it is to do. It will help you to get your blood flowing, get rid of tiredness, anxiety and nervousness to start.

Laying down let your legs fall down naturally and your arms down your side, palms facing up.

Breathe in deeply through your abdomen and think about stretching your limbs out. Pull your shoulders down, your head away from your feet, and so on.

Hold this position for several minutes while quieting your head and focusing on your constant breathing.

After you've finished slowly push yourself into a seated relaxed position and then get yourself up.

THE EASY POSE

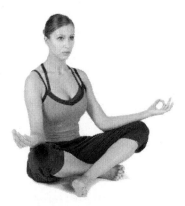

This is a common pose for meditating that normally follows the Corpse. The Easy Pose will help you relax, slow down your metabolism and assist in sitting up straight.

First you will sit your butt down on the ground or yoga mat. Crossing your legs over as you do in grade school, making sure your feet are underneath your knees.

Place your hands on your knees, keeping your back straight and head looking forward.

In this position you will breathe in and out deeply; slowing yourself down into deep inner relaxation.

NECK EXERCISES

The neck area is where a lot of stress, tension and tightness seem to be stored, which can lead to poor posture and even headaches. These exercises will help improve your flexibility, firm up muscles, leaving you loose and relaxed.

Start by dropping your head back gently for a 5 count, then slowly and in a controlled fashion bring it forward so your chin rests on your chest and hold for 5 seconds.

Then looking straight forward with shoulders relaxed and back straight, turn your head as far as you can to the left, so your left ear is over your left shoulder. Hold this for 5 seconds. Do the same thing on the other side.

Repeat these maneuvers and you can even do a full circular motion with your head. Make sure that you do it slowly for effectiveness.

SUN SALUTATION

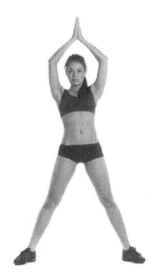

This is a group of twelve exercises that will help you gain strength and become more limber. Along with warming your body up and getting you close to that 6-pack you've always wanted.

1 - Start off in the Yoga Mountain pose. Standing on your mat; just bring both palms to a touching prayer position and breathe out.

2 - While keeping your palms together breathe in and bring your arms straight up above your head towards the ceiling.

3 - Breathe out and fold yourself forward until your hands reach your feet, or as close as you can get.

4 - As you are breathing in, reach your right leg back while arching your back and keeping your head straight and chin forward.

5 - While breathing out move left leg back beside your right into plank position. Here you'll keep your back and legs in a straight line, while placing your weight on your hands and feet.

6 - While holding your breath, bring your knees down, then your chest and forehead, all while making sure your hips are up and toes still curled under.

7 - Now breathe in while stretching forward and bending back. Making sure your arms are straight.

8 - Breathe outward; bring your toes underneath you, pressing your heels to the floor, while sticking your bum and hips up to the ceiling.

9 - Taking a deep breath in, bring your right leg forward into a low lunge position. Make sure the leg extended back has the top of the foot and leg resting on the floor

and your chin is up with your face forward.

10 - Breathing out while you bend forward towards the floor again, until your hands touch your feet.

11 - Breathing in deeply stand in an upright position bringing your arms back behind you, while bending back from the waist.

12 - Breathe out in a controlled fashion, slowly coming back to Tadasana; standing up straight with your arms at your side.

Feels fantastic, doesn't it?

DOUBLE LEG RAISE

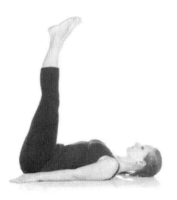

This exercise will help strengthen your core and this is going to help you get strong for numerous other yoga poses.

Start by lying flat on the floor.

Breathe in while raising both legs up, keeping your bum

on the floor and legs straight.

Breathe out while lowering your legs in a controlled fashion to the count of five. Repeat this five to ten times. Keeping in mind it's very important to keep your back on the floor at all times.

As you get stronger you will be able to lower your feet closer to the floor.

STANDING FORWARD BEND

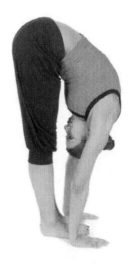

This will give you a great back stretch; both lower and upper. In addition it will work your calf and leg muscles. Here you will stretch out creaks and cracks and loosen up your body. All while relaxing because of increased blood flow to your head.

Stand with arms at your sides. While keeping your back straight bend your knees and gently lean forward so your tummy hits your upper legs. Make sure you keep your back strong so it doesn't sink in.

With your weight on your heels; relax your groin and pelvis area. Don't forget to breathe.

Slowly stretch your head down towards your toes with your chest resting on your legs. Grab your ankles and stretch gently to lengthen yourself.

It's very important to keep your lower back strong because you will lose the purpose of the exercise if it arches on you.

Next you can slowly stand up back to your start position. Ensuring you are breathing from your belly in a controlled fashion.

CAT POSE

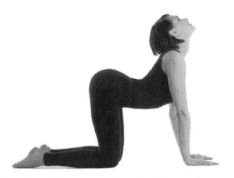

This one helps to align your body, focusing on your core and breathing. It's very energizing when done correctly.

Begin on your hands and knees; just how a cat stands. Your hands should be right under your shoulders and your knees right under your hips. Have your middle finger pointing forward and fingers spread for stability.

Keep your back flat; while looking down at the floor. What this is referred to is the 'neutral' position; where your spine is elongated and relaxed, void of pressure.

Breathing in deeply, and as you exhale turn your hips into the cat tilt. This is done by sucking your tummy in towards the spine. While doing this squeeze your butt, pressing firmly down on your hands so that your shoulders stay up.

Round your spine, push your back up towards the ceiling, while looking down at the floor and curling your head inward.

This will help to loosen your spine and release stress from your back. This also stretches your head, neck, back and shoulders. You will be stimulating your gastrointestinal system and spinal juices, reducing stress and improving circulation.

BOW POSE

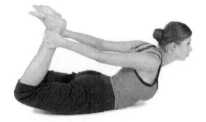

This one will help open your chest and strengthen your back. Working your body differently than it's conditioned to.

First lie on your tummy with your hands at your side and palms facing upward.

Bend your knees and move your heels back toward your butt. Now grab your ankles by reaching behind you. Make sure your weight is on your tummy.

Now gently pull your ankles upward, raising your knees, and feel the stretch further. Make sure you are breathing regularly and focus on it so that your body will naturally relax and you will increase your flexibility.

CHILD'S POSE

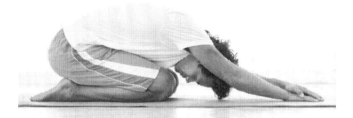

This is a fantastic pose to help your body relax, while stretching out your shoulders and back. It's also used to re-balance you after any sort of backward bend.

It will also help stretch your hips, thighs, lower back and ankles.

To start you can kneel comfortably with your butt resting on your knees and your arms on your lap. Slowly lower your forehead to the floor and then place your arms outstretched in from of you.

Now rest your forehead on the floor and bring your arms back around to your sides with your palms facing up.

PLOUGH POSE

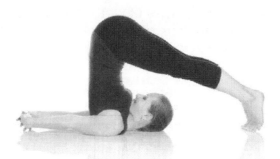

This one will be a little more of a challenge for a beginner. So make sure you are comfortable with yoga before attempting.

Poor posture is an issue at least from time to time with most of us and the Plough pose will help with this.

It will help alleviate soreness and stiffness in your neck and lower back by stretching these muscles and relieving strain. Sounds great to me!

Experts also agree that it helps smooth out digestion, and improve the function of kidneys, your gall bladder and liver.

Start by lying down on your back with your hands straight back behind you, resting on the floor above your head.

Bring your legs straight up to a 90 degree position, legs straight and heels flexed. Don't forget to breathe in through your nose and out through your mouth.

Now boost your hips up off the floor with your abdominals. Continue right on over beyond your head with your legs fairly straight. This now appears that you are folded in half.

Now lift your back up and move your legs past your head and place your toes on the ground. Keep your back solid and straight and gently move your hands back around behind your back.

Place your arms up on your lower back, as close as you care near your shoulder blades. Elbows should ideally be at shoulder width.

As you relax your legs should stretch further and further backwards. Concentrate on your breathing so your muscles will release more.

Slowly bring your legs back to the mat while rolling back down gently, feeling it through your vertebra.

My Thoughts . . .

These are how you execute a few beginner yoga poses. The exciting part is there are hundreds of different poses you can learn. Starting with the basic ones and working your way up as you gain confidence and get more and more comfortable with yoga.

The sky really is the limit and that's the fascinating part. Each new pose helps you to connect your mind and body, while stretching and strengthening your body as a whole.

Need I say more?

Final Thoughts . . .

So what do you think my friends? Are you excited to get started? Please keep in mind that this is just the tip of the mountain when it comes to yoga. Because yoga is one of those things that you will never be able to learn all of it.

You will always be able to better your skills and knowledge and make new discoveries about yourself each and every day. It really is amazing to think about.

Time for you to be united with yourself and your beginner yoga session is your first step in doing this. I hope that you enjoyed all the information and tips outlined in this book. Yoga is definitely a positive aspect of life and it changes the way you feel, the way you look, and the way you react to everyday life. It's made a tremendous difference in my life!

Most of all, I hope that you take action and begin Yoga and start on the road to a better, less stressful and more relaxing life. Good health to you! Thank you for reading!

Printed in Great Britain
by Amazon.co.uk, Ltd.,
Marston Gate.